Sleep, Perchance to Dream

By
Lynne D M Noble

Copyright 2024 Lynne D M Noble

Independently published

Contents

Acknowledgement

I am indebted to all those insomniacs who have discussed the impact that a lack of sufficient good quality sleep has on their lives, with me.

I hope that this book goes some way to finding that elusive pathway to a good night's sleep.

Preface

Sleep is defined as a condition of body and mind which typically recurs for several hours every night, in which the nervous system is inactive, the eyes closed, the postural muscles relaxed, and consciousness practically suspended.

Based on the above definition, it appears that sleep is becoming an elusive commodity nowadays. Very few people do appear to be able to shut themselves off from the day's cares once they climb into bed. Their consciousness is not practically suspended. Things revolve round and round in their head. Their nervous system is far from inactive.

Of course, there are some people who do appear to exist on very little sleep but they are few and far between. Most people appear to complain of not getting enough sleep. They talk of tossing and turning - of finding it difficult to get off to sleep or, once they have drifted off, waking up in the early hours, unable to join the land of slumber once again.

Good quality sleep is absolutely vital to our mental and physical health. Sleep deprivation will affect our relationships and our mood. A poor night's rest means that we will not be able to engage properly with work or significant others the following day. Long term, poor quality sleep, or lack of enough sleep can lead to depression, obesity, diabetes, high blood pressure and heart disease, among others.

When an individual is sleep deprived, the brain reduces a hormone called leptin and raises another called ghrelin. Ghrelin is an appetite stimulant and this offers a potential explanation for the link between sleep and obesity.

Sleep is refreshing and restoring. It is when healing and repair takes place. We cannot ignore this. If we do so, we do so at our peril. Unfortunately, the fast pace of our lives, intrudes into this restorative phase. We find it difficult to wind down or put worries and concerns to one side. Some people appear able to use the time of sleep to problem solve areas of concern, without it affecting their overall health. Others just find their past troubles interfere with their ability to drop off. Their edginess weaves itself into their psyche and appears to serve no useful purpose.

Of course, some people do not appear to have any specific reasons for their sleep difficulties but they are still troubled by sleep deprivation. They may follow good 'sleep hygiene' by not eating a heavy meal late at night, not watching any stimulating programmes or using a screen two hours before bed. They may reduce the temperature of their bedroom a couple of degrees. The reduction in temperature helps our body get ready for sleep. Still, sleep is elusive.

When we look at the quality of sleep, we need to investigate internal and external factors which can negatively affect this essential state. It is possible to be deficient in a nutrient or nutrients which assist the process of sleep. Some people find melatonin useful and others don't. Melatonin is the hormone which regulates sleep. As daylight fades the production of melatonin increases and we feel sleepy. As light increases, the production of melatonin decreases and we wake up. Blue and white light impact mostly on our inability to produce melatonin which is why it is better not to look at screens late at night. However, any chink of light filtering through the window from a street light or from a clock will impact on the production of melatonin. Black out blinds are not a wasted expense when insomnia is a problem.

If supplementation with melatonin does not help insomnia, then clearly the cause is not due to a lack of melatonin. As such further investigation is required into the reason for sleep problems.

It is quite normal to have periods of deep and lighter sleep. Periods of wakefulness do not bother some people but, for others it may. Night time can bring periods of great loneliness and isolation for some people making natural periods of near wakefulness difficult to bear.

When investigating insomnia, the sufferer has to be their own sleuth. With a little detective work, the causes and potential remedies are within their reach. This book is intended to help the individual identify those causes and address them so that the negative impact that sleep deprivation can bring, is brought under control.

About the Author

Lynne Noble was born in 1953 in Huddersfield, West Yorkshire. From a very early age, Lynne showed an interest in nutrition and genetics avidly reading any books that she could get her hands on at the time.

Initially, Lynne studied orthopaedics but events led her to work with the elderly mentally infirm. Here, her interest in neurodegenerative disorders and pain syndromes developed.

Lynne undertook rigorous programmes of study, completing her Cert Ed., (FE) BSc (Hons) and Adv. Dip Education simultaneously before moving onto her M.Ed.

From there she took further demanding programmes in Human Nutrition, Pharmacology, Neuroscience, Genetics and Immunology. During this time, she was given many prestigious awards for her academic work. It was noted then that Lynne was not afraid of tackling difficult subjects.

She began her law degree but ill health prevented her from pursuing this. However, in this time, she moved from being a foster parent to adoptive parent.

She has been instrumental in setting up projects in the community for disadvantaged groups.

She is a member of the Guild of Health Writers.

Now retired, she lives with her husband in a historic Georgian riverside town in the West Midlands. She enjoys gardening, watching her husband bowling and researching.

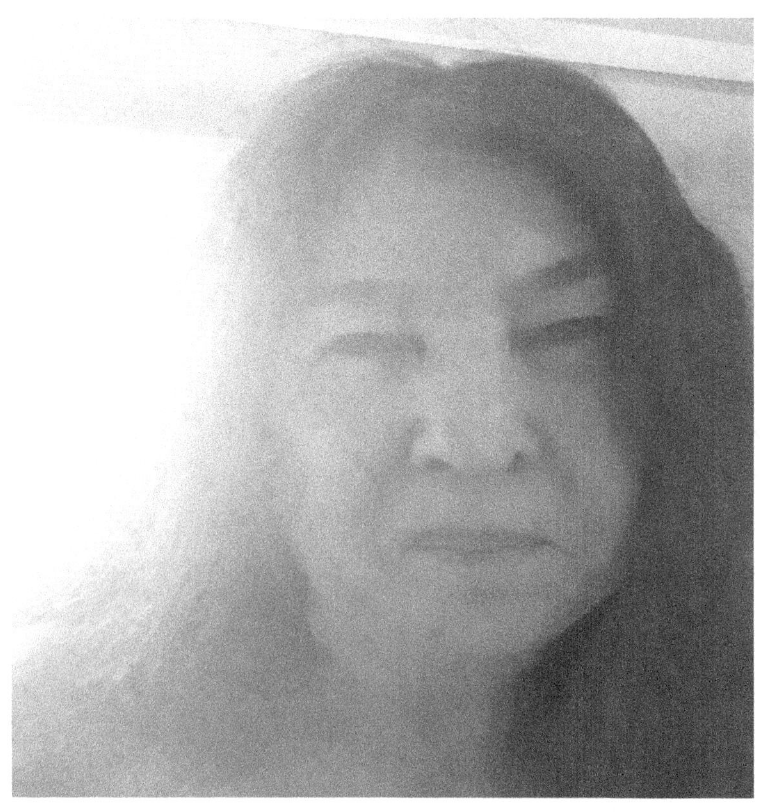

Author Lynne Noble at home

https://quintessentiallylynne.weebly.com/nutritional-medicine.html

Stages of sleep

There are four stages of sleep which need to be passed through before a sleep cycle is completed. Each stage of sleep lasts between 5-15 minutes and the whole sleep cycle – which ends with Rapid Eye Movement (REM) – takes approximately 100 minutes.

At first the REM stages are quite short. They are interspersed with longer periods of deep sleep. As sleep progresses, the REM periods get longer and the deeper periods of sleep get shorter.

Stage 1 is the lightest of sleep. It can be seen in states of drowsiness where the person can be easily woken up. This is the type of sleep often experienced on a warm summer's day, where the heat has a soporific effect and people close their eyes and drift off. Brain wave activity has slowed down and the body is very relaxed. It is not unusual to experience sensations of falling in this stage and some people will experience hypnic jerks.

This is often the stage that most people will experience when they are having a power nap.

Stage 2

This stage enters sleep proper. The person is not easily awakened at this stage. However, the slow moving eye rolls which are also seen at stage one, occur at this stage too.

Brain waves continue to slow but there are bursts of activity known as sleep spindles intermixed with K complexes. These phenomena help to protect the brain from awakening from sleep.

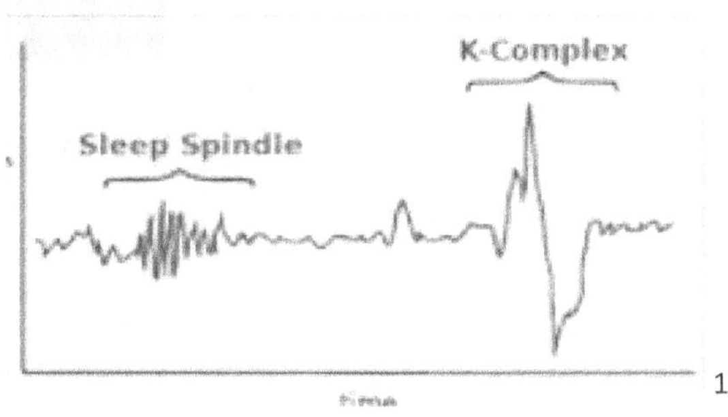

1

Recent research also shows that sleep spindles could be related to your ability to learn. It has been found that the more sleep spindles that were produced in napping, the abler they were to perform learning tasks. Therefore, it appears that too little sleep in stage 2 sleep could impact on your ability to learn and retain knowledge.

Body temperature begins to decrease and the heart rate begins to slow in this stage.

Stage 3

This is the final stage of non REM sleep. It is the most restorative of the stages. It consists of slow waves or delta waves. It is very difficult to awaken someone from this stage of sleep. This is the stage of sleep where the parasomnias occur such as night terrors and sleep walking.

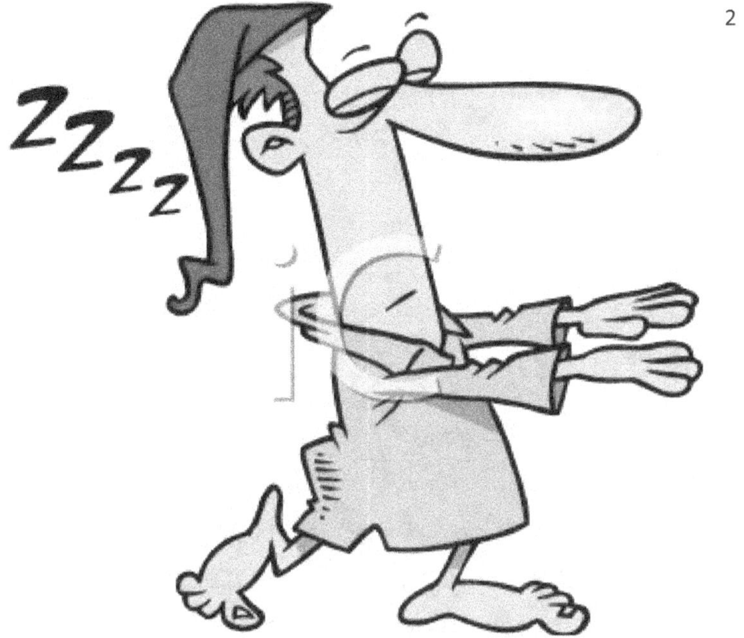

During the deep sleep stage human growth hormone is release and helps repair any damage to your body and muscles. The immune system is also strengthened.[3]

REM sleep

---

[3] http://www.clipartguide.com/_pages/0511-1003-1503-3964.html

This is the stage when dreaming occurs. The eye movements are rapid and move from side to

side. Although it is relatively easy to awaken someone at this stage, the individual will look and feel groggy.

The first three stages of sleep occur **followed by stage one again** before REM sleep occurs. REM sleep is an important stage of sleep for your memory and emotional health. Dreams can help you work through emotional issues and further, help regulate what memories are filed away in short or long term memory.

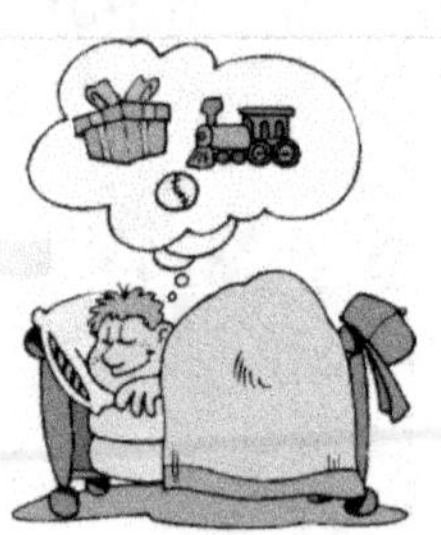

[4]

REM stage of sleep involves dreaming

[4] http://clipart-library.com/clipart/852913.htm

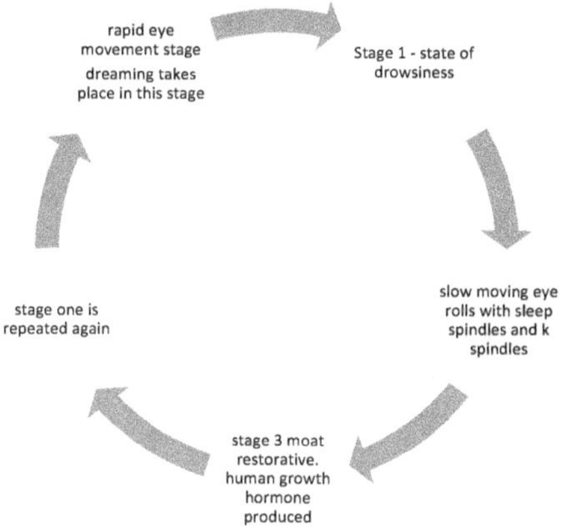

The sleep cycle

The circadian rhythm

The circadian rhythm is a 24-hour internal body clock that controls your sleep-wake cycle. This internal clock is located in a part of the brain known as the hypothalamus.

The hypothalamus is intimately connected with the optic nerves. When these register that it is getting dark and they have passed this information onto the hypothalamus then melatonin will be produced. Melatonin is a

sleep hormone which makes you feel sleepy.
This normally peaks at around 2am.

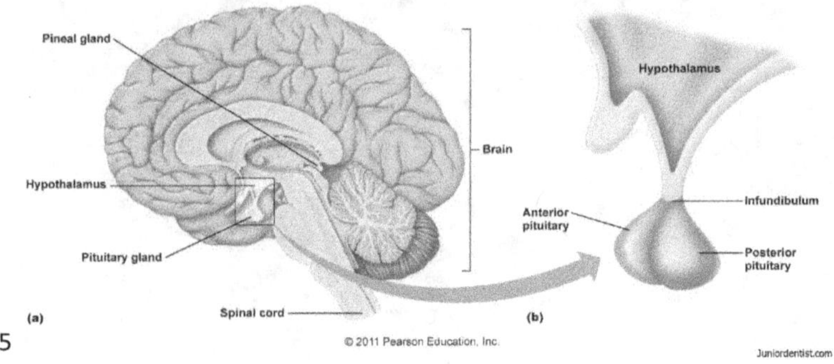

5

The hypothalamus is involved in sleep and melatonin production

A number of common nutrients are needed to aid the optimum working of the sleep cycle.

Vitamin B12 is required for the synthesis of melatonin. It is not surprising that as ageing progresses that levels of vitamin B12 tend to drop. Vitamin B12 needs and acidic environment to be detached from its protein source. Not only does stomach acidity appear to drop as ageing progresses but diets change.

---

[5] https://www.pinterest.co.uk/pin/828803137645771337/?lp=true

Vitamin B12 is found in animal protein. The elderly is less likely to eat meat for a number of reasons.

They find chewing difficult

They can't be bothered now that there is only one person or no family to cook for

It is too expensive to buy on a pension.

Thiamine is also known as vitamin B1 and it is becoming increasingly clear that most people are deficient in it. It has numerous functions in the body including transporting fuel into the cells so that it can be burnt for energy. Not only does this improve energy levels – and mood – enormously so that one is genuinely ready for sleep at night time but it is involved in GABA production.

Studies have shown altered sleeping patterns in the thiamine deficient patient such as fatigue such that sleeping during the day known as 'catnapping' or 'having 40 winks' is rife. Once thiamine is supplemented   then these day bouts of nodding off do not occur.

Gamma-aminobutyric acid (GABA) is found naturally in the brain. It helps induce sleep by reducing anxiety and helping promote relaxation.

The prescription medications Pregabalin and Gabapentin work on this principle.

Nevertheless, these GABA analogues do not work wholly in the same way as the naturally derived GABA. Massive weight gain is associated with prescription medications.

These prescription medications would not be needed if sufficient thiamine and its activating magnesium were found in diets, but both thiamine and magnesium are high in the list of nutrients which are generally deficient in the population as a whole.

GABA supplements in the dosage of 100mg-300mg for sleep latency but these tend to be broken down quickly   and could result in the person taking the supplements waking up in the early hours of the morning.

Stomach upsets, poor balance, double vision and headaches are also side effects.

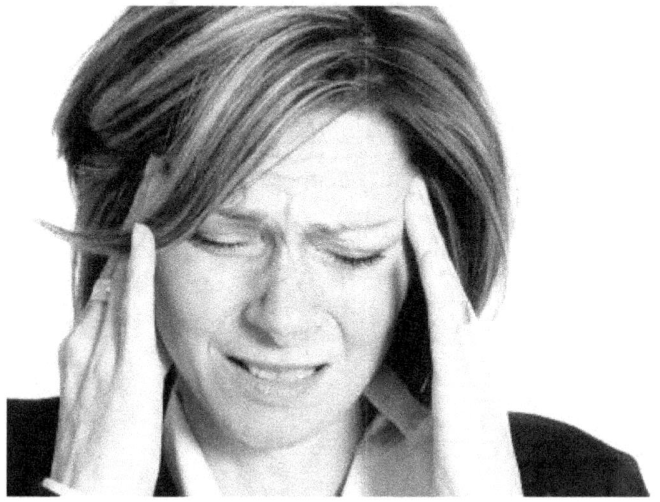

Headaches are a side effect of the prescription GABA analogues.

As daylight approaches, the part of the hypothalamus involved in the sleep wake cycle will trigger the release of cortisol. This will help wake you up.

Cortisol is also released when you are stressed which is why some people toss and turn and cannot get to sleep. The best way, if you are stressed, is to go for a long and uplifting walk. This will use up the hormone that is causing the edginess and thoughts going into overdrive.

When the sleep cycle is disrupted then the immune system dysfunctions. Studies have shown that levels of T cells (white cells) which are important part of the immune system that kill viruses, drop after one good night's sleep is missed.

The circadian rhythm is affected by

- jet lag
- shift work
- social sleeping (having a lie in)
- electronic devices
- The seasons – very short or very long days

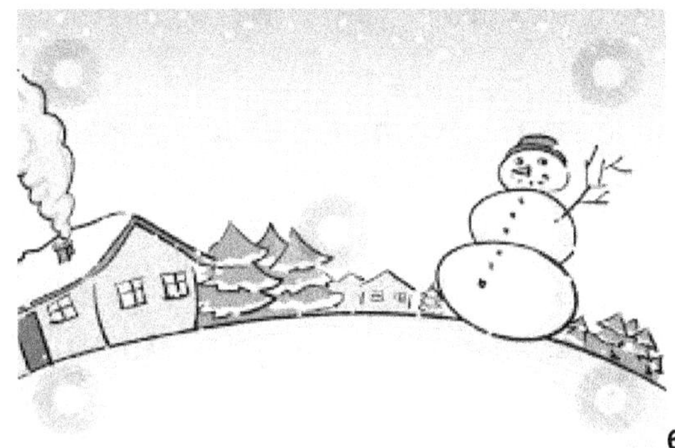

6

Seasonal affective disorder affects sleep patterns as well as mood.

---

[6] http://www.thelockinmovie.com/free-clip-art-winter-scenes/

Sleep Deprivation Due to Pain

There is little doubt that pain is one of the greatest sleep stealers there is. When we talk about pain we are referring to chronic pain or neuropathic pain as opposed to acute pain.

Acute pain is a sharp pain which is felt when we initially injure ourselves. It may occur as a result of standing on a nail or stubbing our toe or trapping our finger in the door. Acute pain is followed by chronic pain which is duller, thudding and more aching. Chronic pain, as its name suggests goes on for a long, long time and often appears to serve no useful purpose.

Painkillers such as paracetamol and ibuprofen - which most people are familiar with – do not work on acute pain. They would not address, for example, the pain of a scalpel – only anaesthetics do this.

Paracetamol, ibuprofen and opioids address chronic pain which are part and parcel of inflammatory conditions such as arthritis or tendonitis.

They can dull the aches and pains of viruses such as colds and 'flu. As such these common painkillers can help someone who has chronic pain, have a good night's sleep but not everyone can take some of these more common painkillers. Those people who are on methotrexate, for example, cannot take non-steroidal anti- inflammatory drugs (NSAID's) such as ibuprofen. NSAID's are associated with allergic reactions. Opioids are well known for their constipating side effects.

Sometimes the negative side effects can outweigh the pain relief that is given.

Paracetamol operates from the central nervous system and ibuprofen from the peripheral nervous system. The combined effects of these two common over the counter medications is greater than the sum of the individual effects. This is fine if the individual can tolerate both but not so good if they cannot. Breakthrough pain is more likely to occur disrupting a good night's sleep.

Ibuprofen is also known to be a risk factor for ulcerations in the digestive tract.

The end product of paracetamol metabolism is phenacetin. Phenacetin was withdrawn decades ago due to its link with dementia.

Vioxx was another popular analgesic which was withdrawn after it was found to cause significant heart problems in those taking it. One study found that 25% of people taking it suffered a heart attack within two weeks of taking it.

Vioxx was also linked to a massive increase in stroke.

Currently, Naproxen is the drug of choice offered on prescription should someone be suffering from chronic pain. The side effects are not acceptable but include;

Blood clots

Bleeding and the potential for anaemia

Fluid retention

Heart attack

Congestive heart failure

 High blood pressure

Kidney or liver disease

Stroke

Hypersensitivity reactions

Dehydration

Which begs the question why the source of the chronic pain is not investigated. Nutritional therapy addresses this very well – and completely – although the full effects of correcting a nutritional deficiency could occur within minutes or take months BUT although the full effect may not be felt for some weeks, there is still some effect building up and without the side effects of the commonly prescribed medications.

Breakthrough pain is pain which occurs between the administrations of regular scheduled painkillers. In some cases, the doses of painkiller can be increased but, in some cases this is not possible without such a move being harmful. Some people may turn to alternative medicine to alleviate breakthrough pain. This may include aromatherapy, acupuncture or massage.

Many amino acids have powerful anti-inflammatory and analgesic properties. They can be used alongside prescribed and over the counter medications as an adjunctive medication although they can just as easily be used as the primary medication.

When breakthrough pain occurs the adjunctive treatments we can use safely without reducing any prescribed or over the counter medications are easily obtainable. They can make a whole world of difference in the search for a good night's sleep. The main ones are:

 Anti- Histamines such as Cetirizine 10mg which is obtainable from supermarkets at low prices. The supermarkets own brand is just as good as the more expensive branded ones.

Most people associate anti-histamines such as the sedating ones like Cetirizine with allergies and they would be correct in doing so. However, anti-histamines have an anti-inflammatory action and, as such, the ability to reduce pain.

However, antihistamines should never be taken for more than a few days as they reduce the effectiveness of the immune system to combat infection.

Histamine is a vaso-active amine which has an important role in the initial acute inflammatory response. It is stored in mast cells, basophils and platelets. Histamine is released from cells by stimuli which include substances involved in acute inflammation.

Histamine increases vasodilation – that is, it widens blood vessels. It also makes them more permeable too. Histamine is a chemical mediator and brings immune system substances to the site of injury. The swelling and other substances irritate pain receptors causing pain.

Histamine is certainly implicated in joint pain.

There is also a condition known as histamine intolerance which has the potential to disrupt sleep. Within the brain histamine is responsible for regulating the sleep-wake cycle. If too little histamine is available, then excessive sleepiness can occur. In contrast, too much histamine can lead to insomnia.

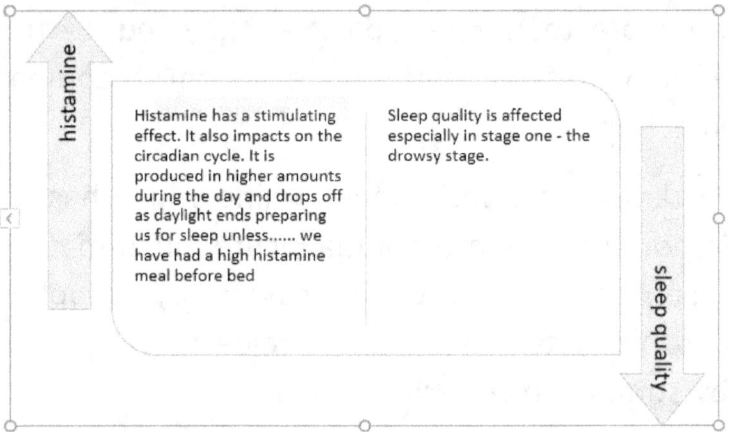

Histamine also had an impact on the biological clock – our circadian rhythm – which tells us when to eat and when to sleep or wake up. As histamine is stimulating and suppresses sleep then it is wise to avoid foods containing high amounts of histamine and high histamine releasing foods near to bed time.

Alcohol is often drunk before bedtime as a relaxant. However, alcohol is not only high in histamine but it also blocks the enzyme DAO which is important for breaking down histamine.

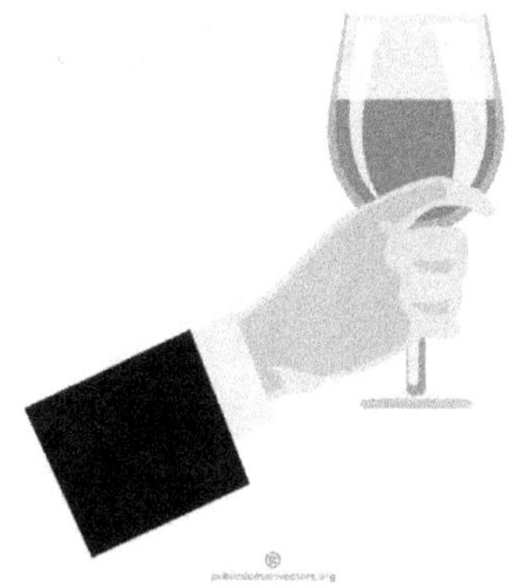

⁷

Diamine oxidase (DAO) is the major enzyme involved in histamine metabolism. It ensures that there is the correct level of histamine available required for the balance of numerous chemical reactions taking place in the body.

---

⁷ https://publicdomainvectors.org/en/free-clipart/Glass-of-wine/51352.html

It does however, require the presence of zinc and magnesium in sufficient quantities to be able to function properly.

DAO also degrades any extracellular (free) histamine which might have occurred through diet or from allergy induced processes in the body.

Olive oil has been found to release DAO into the bloodstream by up to 500%[8]

---

[8] Wollin, A, wang, X, Tso, P. (2017) Nutrients regulate diamine oxidase release from intestinal mucosa). The American Physiological Society, 20, 220

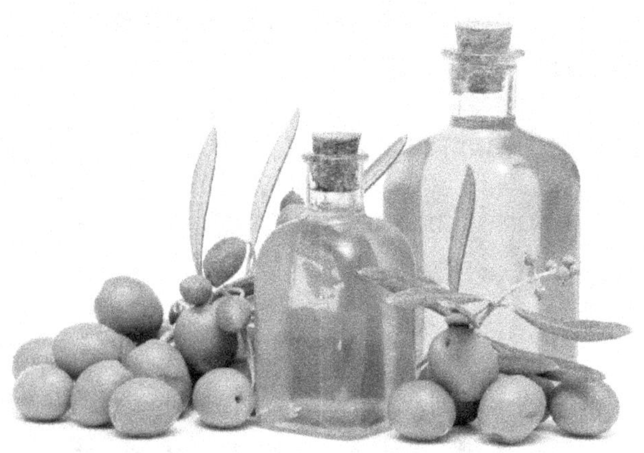

Anti-histamines also counteract high histamine levels and thus have the potential to markedly reduce pain. They are relatively free from side effects. They do have anti-cholinergic effects – that is they have a drying effect which is useful for allergies – and as such can cause constipation in susceptible people -but not to the same degree that opioids do.

As the prime aim of taking anti-histamines is to enable a good night's rest by reducing pain then clearly the sedating antihistamines are the best

---

9 https://oliviaevoo.com/product/arbequina/

ones. They should be taken half an hour before going to bed.

Sedating antihistamines include:

- Chlorphenamine (Piriton)
- Hydroxyzine
- promethazine

Look for over the counter medications which contain one of the above. Piriton, while effective, is short acting – about 4 hours - and may not be suitable for people who have a habit of waking up in the middle of the night. However, there is no reason why another tablet cannot be taken at this point.

Although Cetirizine hydrochloride is supposed to be a non-sedating antihistamine, most people report that it gives them the best pain free, restful night. As always, different products will suit different people. Fortunately, anti-histamines are not expensive which makes the trial and error approach affordable.

Sedating anti-histamines are useful in the short term for anxiety.

What can we use instead of antihistamines to reduce histamine and alleviate chronic pain? Quite simply, vitamin C is far more effective taken in therapeutic doses of 1gram to 2 grams in reducing histamine than any over the counter or prescription medication.

Further, it addresses inflammatory conditions and can help to resolve joint inflammation - and thus pain. It can have a marked effect by   day three although when it comes to repairing the damage done to joints – and which is causing the chronic pain – it needs about 3 months.

Much of the extensive bruising that the elderly appears to suffer from after having a tiny knock will be due to the fragility of their blood vessels brought about by vitamin C insufficiency.

Indeed, research shows that vitamin C insufficiency ranks fourth of nutrient deficiency in the United States.

The recommended intake of 75mg for adult females and 90mg daily for adult males is far too low to bring about optimum health. These levels were introduced as preventing scurvy.

People then took it that this was sufficient for the running of all they systems in the body when it is not. If you have any condition ending in 'itis' then you have greatly increased need for vitamin C.

Current recommended levels which are more realistic are at least 450mg daily.

Neutrophils are immune system cells which are a first line of defence when infection strikes. They are activated by vitamin C. Studies have shown that at the first sign of infection neutrophils cannot be activated because vitamin C levels drop rapidly. It is recommended that 3g (3000mg) of vitamin C is taken for the first three days of any infection).

Vitamin C does not store well at all. It is unlikely that there is much vitamin C in the fruit and vegetables that have been transported halfway around the world and then lain in the supermarket waiting to be bought They may look good but....

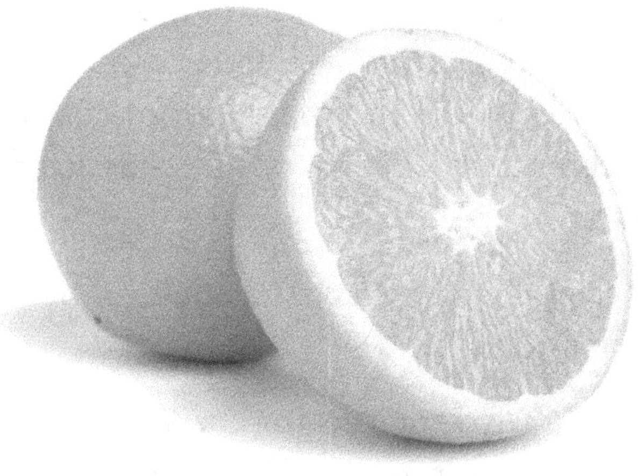

There may not be as much vitamin C in oranges as you have been led to believe. Storage and sunlight destroy vitamin C very quickly

Magnesium as an analgesic

Magnesium is a mineral that's crucial to the body's function. Magnesium helps keep blood pressure normal, bones strong and the heart rhythm steady. It also aids sleep.

More and more the benefits of magnesium in relieving pain and inflammation are becoming clear. Studies have found that, at the cellular level magnesium reduces inflammation. It was found that when an inflammatory condition is produced then a magnesium deficiency is created.

Increasing magnesium intake decreases inflammation.

Magnesium is required for the activity of over 700 enzyme systems in the body. There are a number of ways in which magnesium reduces pain and inflammation. For example, magnesium is a natural calcium channel blocker. Excessive calcium is one of the most pro-inflammatory substances that there is.

The ratio of calcium to magnesium has always held to be that of twice the amount of calcium - 800mg daily – to half that of magnesium – 400mg. More recent studies have argued that the daily intake of these minerals should be equal. It may be that the milky drink (which contains calcium) taken at night to enhance sleep has the potential to increase pain!

Research has shown that magnesium can be effective in both muscle and nerve pain.

It is well known that magnesium eases muscle pain by its muscle relaxing abilities. It is these properties which are harnessed in the Epsom salt type bath.

A study on rats which appeared in the *Journal of Physiology* confirmed that magnesium decreases nerve pain.

N-methyl-D-aspartate (NMDA) is a pain carrying neurotransmitter. When this neurotransmitter is stimulated it is a major mechanism of pain.

Some drugs such as Amantadine and Ketamine which help decrease and balance this neurotransmitter have significant side effects. For example, some of the side effects of Amantadine are listed as being
- Depression, anxiety and irritability
- Hallucinations and confusion
- Anorexia

- Dry mouth
- Constipation
- Somnolence
- agitation

among many others.

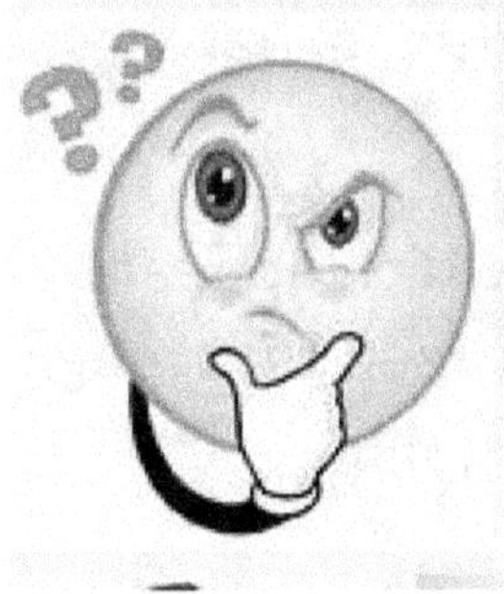

Confusion is a sign of some pain killers

However, magnesium has been found to calm down NMDA without the side effects that most of the prescription drugs have.

The authors of the above study have argued that magnesium deficiency can be a major amplifier of pain and have highlighted that most people are magnesium deficient.

Magnesium deficiency is caused through three main routes. Firstly, a poor diet which lacks green leafy vegetables and nuts may cause low levels of magnesium. However, other culprits are the use of diuretics and laxatives which deplete potassium. When potassium levels are low they automatically deplete the levels of magnesium.

High potassium foods are most fruits – especially bananas – beetroot and meat.

The only contraindication to supplementing with magnesium is for those who have kidney disease

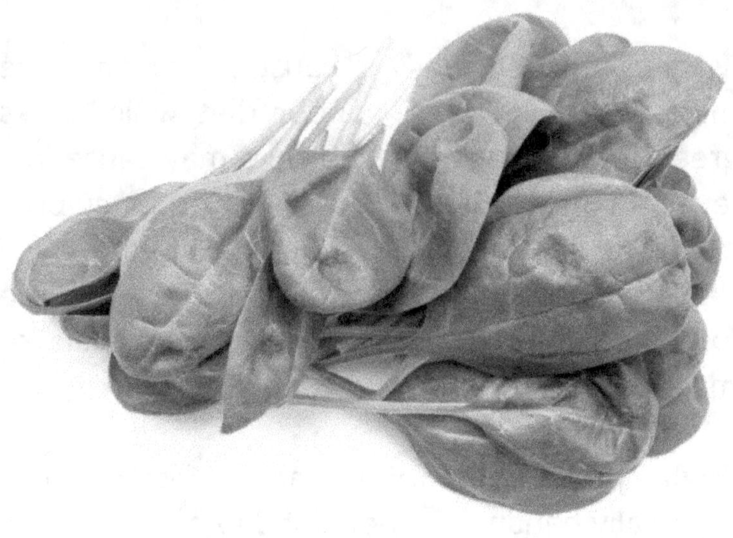

Spinach is a good source of magnesium. Eat your greens is wise advice

Magnesium supplementation for migraine

Magnesium oxide is often used to prevent migraine at a dose of 500mg daily. Evidence for magnesium's effectiveness is in patients who have had aura with their migraines where it is thought that magnesium may prevent waves of brain signalling. These waves –cortical spreading depression – initiate the visual and sensory changes associated with aura.

Magnesium also decreases the release of substance P and glutamate as well as preventing the narrowing of brain blood vessels caused by the neurotransmitter serotonin.

Substance P and glutamate are pain transmitting chemicals.
Substance P is released from the ends of specific sensory nerves and is found in the central and peripheral nervous system. It is associated with inflammatory processes and pain.

Neuronal substance P is stored in vesicles and released when it comes into contact with
- leukotrienes
- prostaglandins
- histamine

among others

From the information we already have we can see that magnesium in conjunction with an antihistamine has the potential to relieve pain.

However, magnesium's sleep inducing qualities aren't just related to its pain relieving capabilities. Magnesium also helps to activate the parasympathetic nervous system which is the system responsible for making you feel calm and relaxed.

Magnesium helps regulate the hormone melatonin which is implicated in the sleep wake cycle.

Secondly, this mineral binds to gamma-butyric acid (GABA) receptors. GABA is the neurotransmitter responsible for calming down nerve activity. As such magnesium is helpful in preparing the body for sleep.

Studies. in mice. have shown that too high or too low a level of magnesium can cause troubled sleep.

People who are more likely to suffer from magnesium deficiency are:

- people on diuretics or laxatives

- people with digestive diseases which affects absorption of nutrients
- people with diabetes as insulin resistance and diabetes are linked with excess magnesium loss
- people who drink a lot of alcohol
- older adults have less magnesium in their diets and are also less efficient at absorbing it.

Magnesium also helps you achieve a deep and restful sleep which can be found in stage three of the sleep cycle.

In a study, elderly participants were given 500mg of magnesium or a placebo. Those taking the magnesium had a better quality of sleep. This group also had higher levels of renin and melatonin. These substances help regulate sleep. [10]

---

[10] https://www.ncbi.nlm.nih.gov/pubmed/23853635

Another study, in mice, found that a magnesium deficiency resulted in sleep patterns that were light and restless.[11]

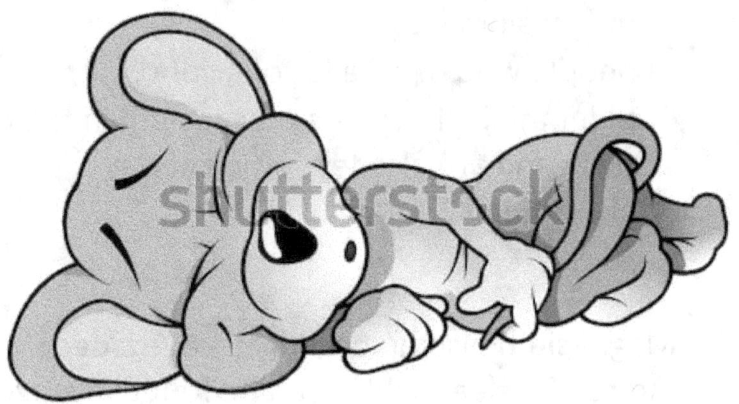

---

[11]https://www.ncbi.nlm.nih.gov/pubmed/8232845

DL Phenylalanine – this essential amino acid has been well researched and documented and is effective in the control of chronic and acute pain syndromes which include

- lower back pain

- osteoarthritis

- joint pain resulting from rheumatoid arthritis

- migraine

- neuralgia

among others

DLPA appears to focus on chronic pain only. It protects the brain own natural endorphins allowing them to continue to act effectively and for longer periods than that of pharmaceutical products.

DLPA has also been found to have strong antidepressant action and is effective in relieving anxiety.

Good sources of phenylalanine are animal foods and beans and nuts.

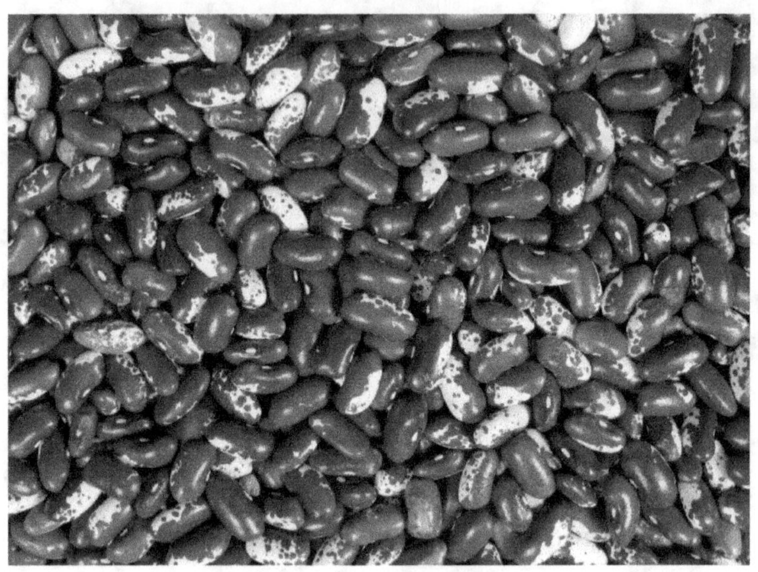

Beans are a good source of phenylalanine

During illness, when appetite is lost and phenylalanine levels are also below optimum levels, then pain is likely to increase. Phenylalanine supplementation should be considered at this time and is available in powdered form and is obtainable from health food shops or online.

Dosage initial dosage would be 2000mg increasing to no more than 4,500mg by two weeks. It is a good adjunctive therapy but can also be used alone.

Amino acids should always be taken on an empty stomach to maximise absorption. In free form they need no digesting and so can act within minutes – far quicker than prescribed medications unless they are the injectable form.

Glutamine is found in muscles. It is known as brain fuel as it easily passes through the blood brain barrier. Glutamine increases the amount of GABA – another amino acid and neurotransmitter – which inhibits pain.

Gkutamine is the amino acid found in the intestinal gut lining and helps conditions such as Crohn's disease, leaky gut syndrome and irritable bowel syndrome. Thus it helps address gut related pain and any damage caused by NSAID's such as ibuprofen.

The best dietary sources are animal protein since animal proteins contains all the essential amino acids. However, also included are:

Grains like oats wheat and rice

Plant based proteins like nuts and legumes

Vegetables with good sources being corn, potatoes, spinach and cabbage

Fermented foods

L glutamine is a conditionally essential amino acid which means that at times of illness, infection or injury much higher amounts than that taken in food on a daily basis are needed.

The body's two primary pain modulators

The body has its own analgesic system which are the neurotransmitters. The two main ones are derived from amino acids

- Gamma amino butyric acid (GABA)

- Endorphins

It is perhaps no surprise that one of these precursor amino acids is DL phenylalanine. Seymour Ehrenpreis PhD., pharmacology professor at Chicago Medical School demonstrated that this endorphinase[12] allowed the medical school to significantly reduce the amounts of opiate medication administered.

Phenylalanine is also useful in reducing food cravings and can assist in weight loss.

---

[12] inhibits the breakdown of pain reliving endorphins

GABA

GABA is a major inhibitory neurotransmitter and helps calm pain and relieve anxiety. It is also an amino acid in its own right. For a long time GABA was not thought capable of crossing the blood brain barrier but more recently evidence has been found for the presence of a GABA transporter in the blood brain barrier. This demonstrates that GABA can enter or exit the brain.

A lack of inhibition by neurotransmitters – mainly GABA – is responsible for many pain states. Some GABA analogues such as Gabapentin and Pregabalin act by inhibiting ion channels which contributes to their analgesic effects.

Glutamine is a precursor to GABA and is easily obtainable from foods such as

- Meat

- Seafood

- Milk

- Nuts

- Eggs

- Cabbage

- Beans

During times of stress, illness and injury – as glutamine is a conditional amino acid – and as the requirement for this amino acid is more than the body can make, supplements may be useful at this point.

Supplements can be bought from health food stores and come in a tablet or powder form. The powder is tasteless and can be sprinkled into soups or over a meal.

L-theanine is another amino acid which is able to increase the levels of GABA.   L-theanine has very few sources and these include tea – both green and black – and mushrooms.

L-theanine differs to that of other amino acid based pain relievers in that it does not induce sleepiness or cause weight gain. Indeed, one of the delightful side effects of L-theanine is that it reduces pain and anxiety while maintaining and promoting alertness.

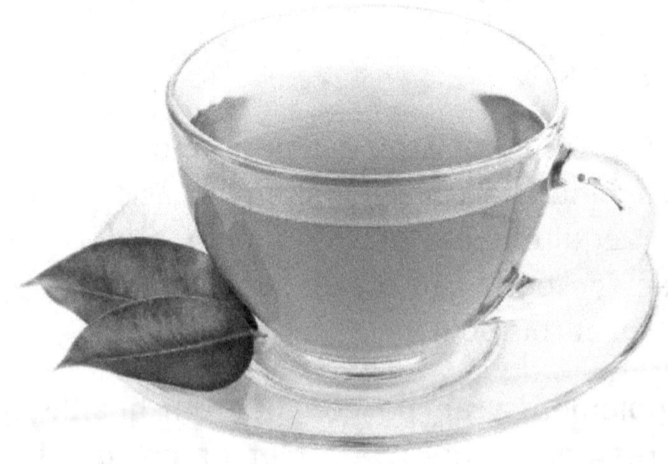

Green tea contains L-theanine

Calcium needs vitamin D to balance it otherwise it can cause pain.

There are quite a number of studies which show increased risks for heart attack and stroke among men and women who supplement with calcium of 1,000 to 1,200mg daily.

It is highly likely that without adequate vitamin D to absorb it, calcium will settle in the arteries instead of the bones where it will help form plaques in the brain and heart.

Extra calcium can also settle in the joints causing joint pain. Further, excessive calcium can cause abdominal and muscle pain, mood disorders and kidney stones.

Further, calcium levels have been found to be higher during deep sleep such as that found in the Rapid Eye Movement phase.

A lack of calcium is a risk factor for disturbed sleep whether this is repeated waking or just finding it difficult to drop off in the first place.

Lower levels of calcium are also associated with night time trips to the toilet.

When calcium levels are insufficient then slow wave activity is also disrupted.

Good sources of calcium are milk and cheese.

A milky drink at bedtimes offers great hope for a good night's sleep for not only does it contain good amounts of calcium but an amino acid called tryptophan.   I shall return to this remarkable amino acid later.

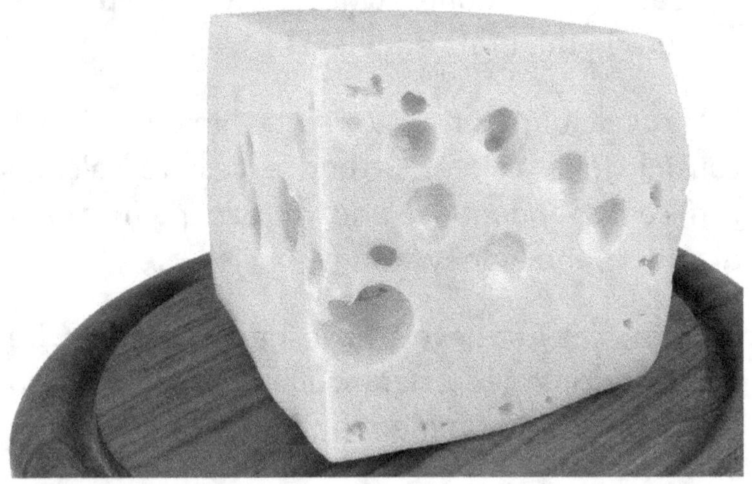

Cheese is a good source of calcium

Glycine is the smallest molecule of those found in the amino acids. It is a non-essential inhibitory amino acid whose inhibitory actions are found in the brain stem and spinal cord. It also has several functions in the central nervous system. Studies[13] have shown that it has a role to play in sleep initiation and maintenance. It is also able to reduce pain and anxiety.

Low dose glycine at a dose of 3g daily prior to going to bed was found to subjectively improve sleep quality. Further, it was also found to reduce sleepiness and fatigue during the day in individuals with insomniac tendencies or restricted sleep time.[14]

Studies also show that there is a relationship between the timing of sleep and core body temperature. The core body temperature will lower at night and induce sleep. Glycine helps in this process.

Conversely, a heavy meal before bed time will increase core body temperature and delay the initiation of sleep.

---

[13] https://www.ncbi.nlm.nih.gov/pmc/articles/PMC4397399/
[14] Bannai *et al*, 2012; Inagawa *et al*,

Similarly, a room which is too warm will also delay the onset of sleep as will a raised body temperature which may happen at time of illness. It is the dip in body temperature which signals the body to make melatonin which encourages us to enter the sleep cycle.

Glycine is found in gelatinous food such as jelly or the meats which need long stewing and whose gravy will form a gelatinous mass when cooled.

Bone broth is especially useful if you are wanting to raise levels of glycine. 25% glycine is found in gelatine.

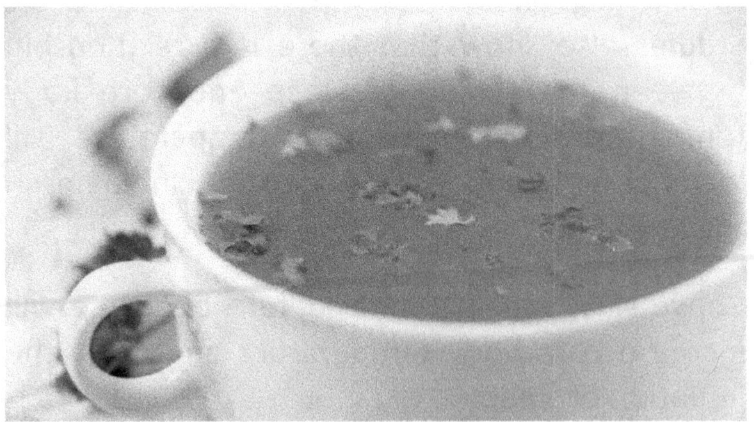

Bone broth; an excellent source of glycine.

Capsaicin, a compound found in chilli peppers, may also raise core body temperature and disrupt sleep. On the other hand, it blocks Substance P which is known to increase pain.

Taking a warm bath or shower may also delay sleep in some individuals where the core body temperature is too high but, in some individuals, a warm bath or shower is relaxing and may aid sleep.

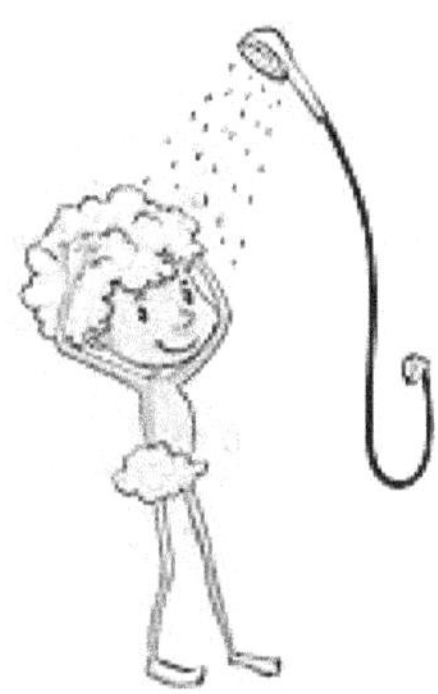

Leg cramps and restless legs appear to be more prevalent as age progresses. My husband, who is in his seventies, has a tendency to jump out of bed double quick at least a couple of times a week complaining of cramps.

Restless legs syndrome appears to be a chronic condition which impacts greatly on sleep quality. It is not painful in the way that leg cramps are and it is perhaps for this reason that it is not given the attention it deserves. Most people are expected to learn to live with it.

Leg cramps can be treated in a number of ways. Some of the remedies can also be tried on restless legs syndrome even though the underlying reason for the symptoms are different. These can include

- Calf stretching exercises before bed

- Taking a sachet of electrolyte solution

- Drinking a small amount of low sodium vegetable juice

- Take a vitamin B complex vitamin – this should be taken in the morning as this vitamin complex helps to release energy

- Take 500mg of magnesium

I am of the opinion that the magnesium, vegetable juice or sachet of electrolytes will be most useful. I have noted that the majority of people with restless legs syndrome are taking diuretics or laxatives and are highly likely to be potassium and magnesium deficient.

Clearly, sleep deprivation needs to be investigated thoroughly in order to establish for the reason for it and, just as importantly, the solution to it.

Some of these symptoms are seen a couple of decades before the symptoms of Parkinson's disease lead to a diagnose of this condition, in which steps can be taken to prevent further deterioration before it manifests itself in other ways. Constipation, which has troubled the sufferer for what is often years, is symptom which precedes full blown Parkinson's disease by many years.

However, for most people, the jerks and restlessness are symptomatic of nutritional deficiencies which can easily be corrected.

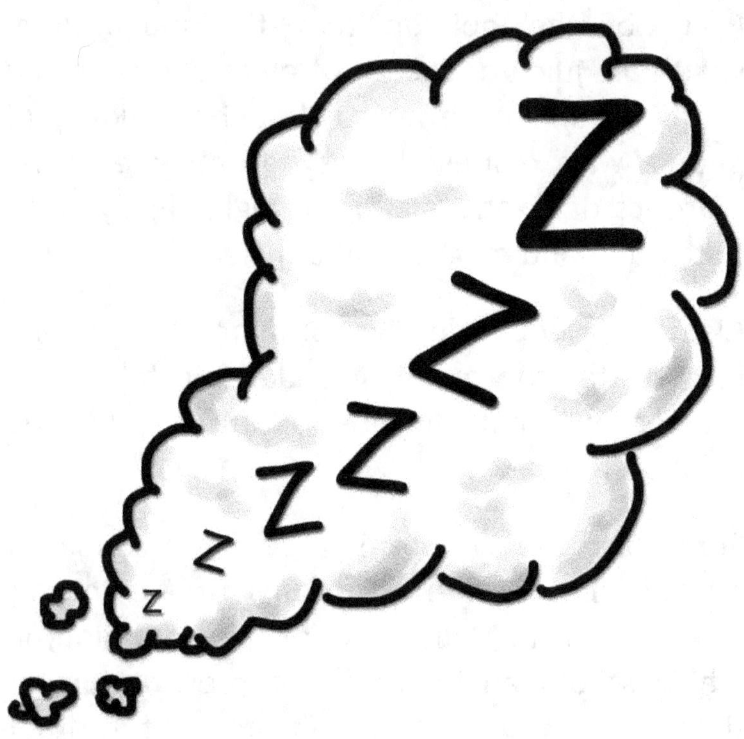

Gastro-oesophageal reflux disorder, indigestion and heartburn.

Indigestion is a vague feeling of discomfort in the chest or upper abdomen. It generally occurs after eating a heavy or high fat meal and can cause bloating and a feeling of fullness. The burning sensation that you sometimes feel in the throat or chest is known as heartburn.

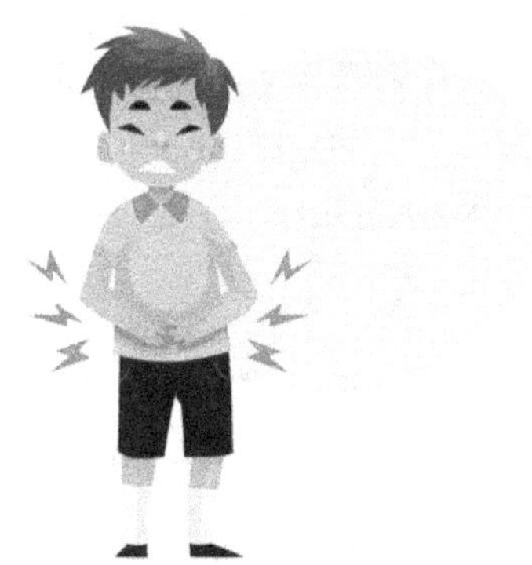

When heartburn occurs more than twice a week then it is considered to be gastro-oesophageal disease (GERD or GORD). This can eventually lead to more serious health problems and/or be a sign of more serious health problems.

There are a number of causes of indigestion which may surprise you. One of these is the addition of niacin to breakfast cereals and similar.

Niacin can be very hard on the stomach and be a risk factor for bleeding and ulceration of the stomach lining.

That cereal snack that you have before bedtime with a cup of hot milk may not be the best for you. However, if you do have symptoms of indigestion and heartburn then take about 20mg of zinc should sort the problem out.

Doctors tend to prescribe PPI's like Lansoprazole. PPI's reduce the acidity in the stomach which prevents you absorbing many of the nutrients you require for good sleep. Some of these nutrients include:

Vitamin B12

Zinc

magnesium

Lifestyle changes are indicated here especially as indigestion has the potential to disrupt sleep. These lifestyle changes include.

- Lose weight; abdominal obesity pushes the contents of the stomach upwards into the gullet

- Eat smaller, more frequent meals, avoid late night snacks and high fat foods. High fat foods take more digesting and can slow down the passage of food from the stomach to the intestines.

- Find the foods triggering the indigestion. Chocolate is a common one. This is likely to be because chocolate increases histamine levels.

- Take exercise about one hour after eating, this will help the food pass from the stomach to the colon.

- Sleep propped up. This prevents gastric juices from backing up into the oesophagus. To achieve this propping up you can either use extra pillows or place a brick under the bed legs at the head end.

- Don't smoke or drink alcohol. Nicotine relaxes the sphincter muscle at the end of the oesophagus so that the contents of the stomach are more likely to back up. Smoking also stimulates stomach acid.

There are a number of medications which can help

Some of the many over the counter remedies include calcium carbonate tablets. These are reasonably effective but if you have pain then increasing calcium may not be the best way forward.

Calcium carbonate is basically chalk. It needs a good acidic stomach in order for it to be absorbed. Calcium citrate, on the other hand, does not need the stomach to be acidic to aid its absorption.

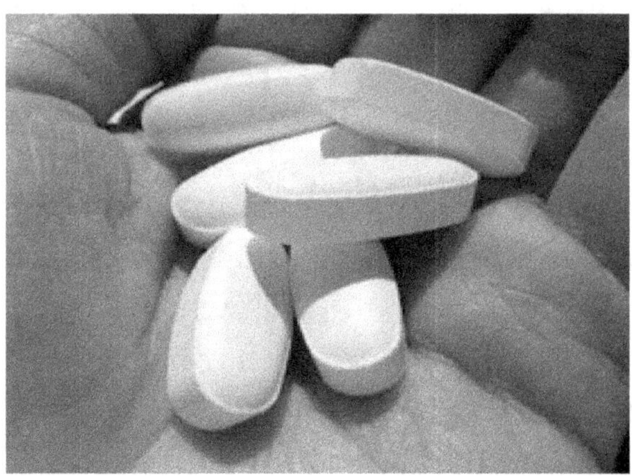

Calcium citrate is far more absorbable than calcium carbonate

Magnesium is good at neutralising acid and can be used as it is found in magnesium supplements. The potential for magnesium to neutralise acid is harnessed in the proprietary treatment Milk of Magnesia.

Histamine Receptor Antagonists such as Zantac and Pepcid AC are useful as are Proton Pump inhibitors. However, they do have side effects and should never be considered for long term use. The reduction in stomach acidity will allow pathological bacteria to flourish. As we have already discussed nutrients such as Vitamin B12 requires an acidic environment before it can be separated from its source and be used in the body.

I have found antihistamines to be just as useful for ameliorating the effects of indigestion as any of the recommended medications produced especially for acid indigestion. However, given the concerning side effects of antihistamines such as profound weight gain and an increased risk of infection, I would not recommend if vitamin C was handy since this is far better at stabilising mast cells without the unwanted side effects that proprietary antihistamines have.

Some pro-kinetics like Prucolapride help propel the stomach contents on so that it empties faster. However, eating dark green leafy vegetables are just as effective.

Almonds are an old fashioned treatment for GORD. Six almonds taken as soon as the symptoms manifest themselves often deals effectively with this condition.

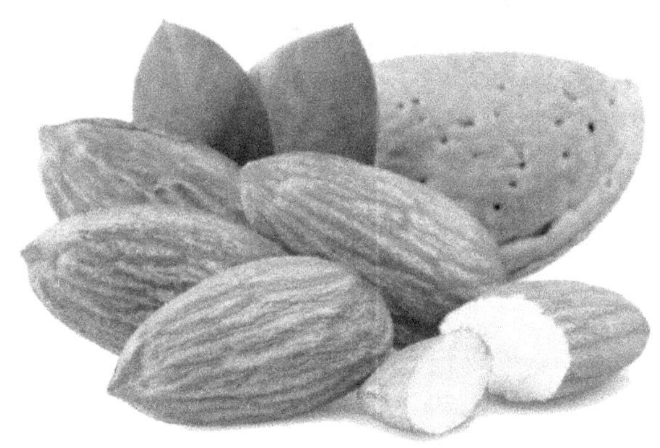

Eating 6 almonds is an old fashioned treatment for GORD

Almonds help neutralise stomach acid as does banana and oatmeal.

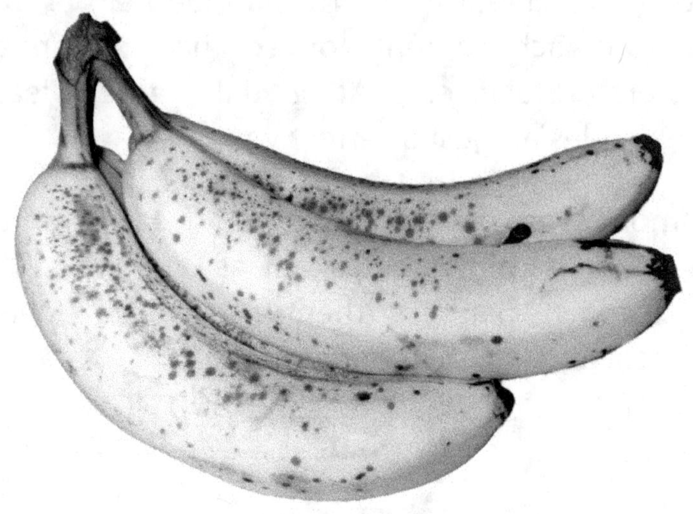

Bananas help to neutralise stomach acid

Foods, supplements and others which aid sleep

There are a great many foods and supplements which will aid sleep. Some you will be familiar with and some you may not have heard of or thought of as sleep inducing agents.

L-tryptophan is an amino acid. It is an essential amino acid because the body cannot make it and it must be acquired from food. It goes without saying that a good diet is vital if we are to solve some of the sleep problems that exist nowadays.
Some great sources of tryptophan are:

- Eggs
- Pineapples
- Cream cheese
- Salmon
- Nuts and seeds
- turkey
- oats
- lentils

When L-tryptophan is absorbed from food it is converted to 5-HTP and from then on to serotonin, melatonin or nicotinamide – otherwise known as vitamin B6.

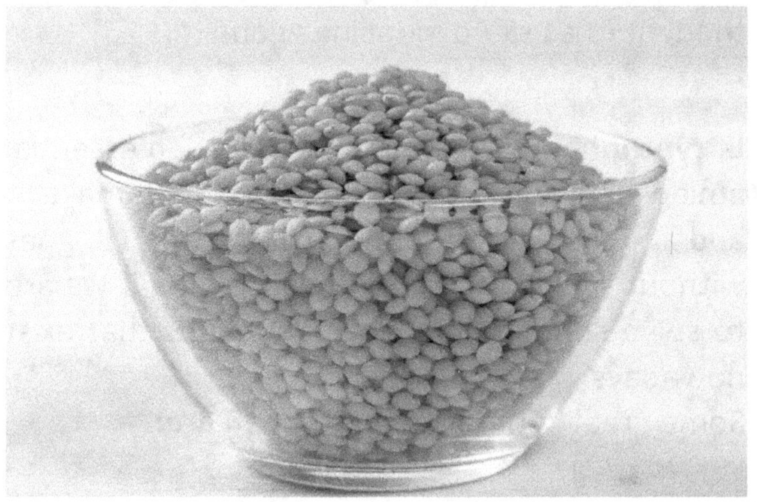

Lentils contain good amounts of the amino acid tryptophan which is a sleep inducer

One of the functions of serotonin is that it can cause blood vessels to narrow. It has been thought to be implicated in the instigation of migraine and it can alter mood.

Serotonin's main functions, however, are to transmit signals between nerve cells and it is also used in the manufacture of melatonin – the sleep hormone.

 Eating carbohydrates make tryptophan available to the brain which is one of the reasons we can feel sleepy after eating a carbohydrate loaded meal.

Cherries are a natural source of melatonin. Drinking tart cherry juice has been found to be beneficial in improving sleep duration and quality.

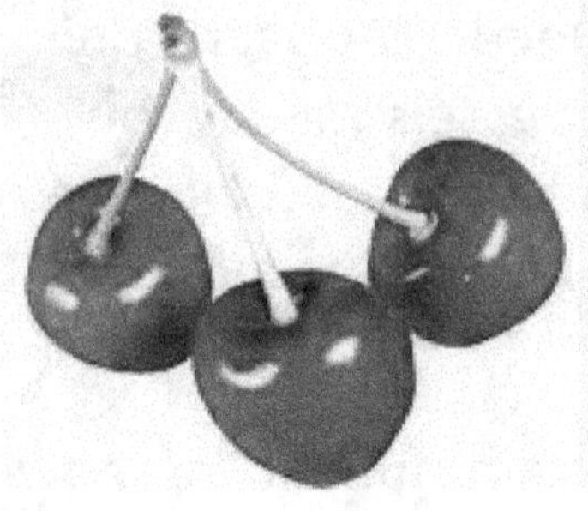

Cherries contain melatonin and so aid sleep

Other good sources of melatonin are

- corn, asparagus, tomatoes, pomegranate, olives, grapes broccoli and cucumber

- rice, barley, rolled oats

- Nuts and seeds such as sunflower seeds, peanuts, walnuts, flaxseed and walnuts.

However, garbanzo beans are invaluable in that they are loaded with free tryptophan. This means it is not attached to a protein as it is in other foods. This makes the uptake of this source of tryptophan the best that there is.

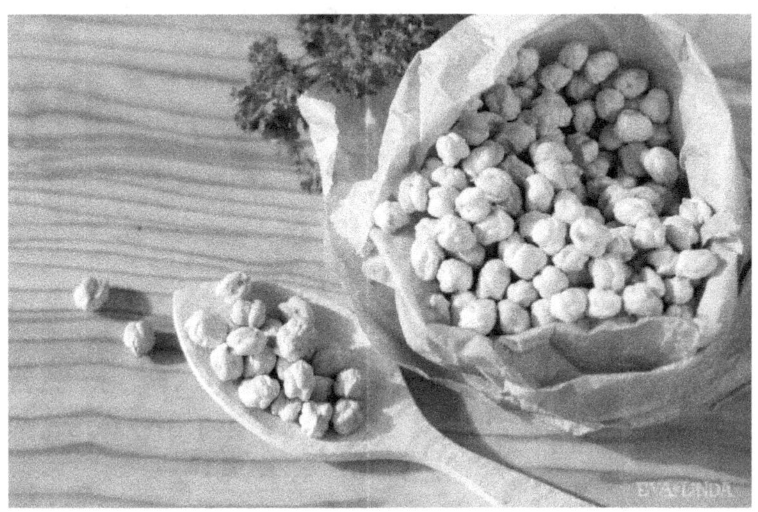

Garbanzo beans are a source of free tryptophan. As well as aiding sleep they would be an effective treatment for migraine.

We could harness this knowledge better if we sat down and thought about it. Clearly heavy meals are not to be recommended before bedtime purely because they raise core body temperature, probably contain fat and hardly allow the body to relax when it is busy digesting. The colon normally rests when the individual is sleeping and is roused into action when the individual wakes up to start a new day. It does not really want its cycle disrupting by late night snacking.

A nightcap full of calcium and raising the levels of tryptophan (which is found in milk)- an hour before bedtime - will do no harm.

One of the best ways of increasing tryptophan is by eating a small dish of lentils and brown rice. Further benefits which they provide are, that as they are complex carbohydrates, they avoid that state of low blood sugar which often affects many people during the early hours and which causes them to wake.

Many people keep a biscuit and a drink at their bedside for times such as this and can settle down after their early morning snack. However, it is preferable if this can be avoided altogether. Biscuits can cause a rapid spike in blood sugar levels which can also disrupt sleep.   Keeping thiamine levels at optimum levels would avoid this.

I mention lentils in particular as lentil soup used to be a particular favourite in the post war years. I had a lot of it when I was a child and continued to make it when I grew up and had a family of my own. I did notice that, when I had friends around, if I served them lentil soup, they tended to complain that they could not stay awake. When this had happened more times than I could recall, I realised that lentils had some soporific inducing qualities.

It worked a treat on the children who slept soundly even on Christmas Eve when excitement would normally keep a child awake most of the night. Rice has similar qualities but lentil soup is far superior. If I was to recommend a night cap, then this is my favourite one.

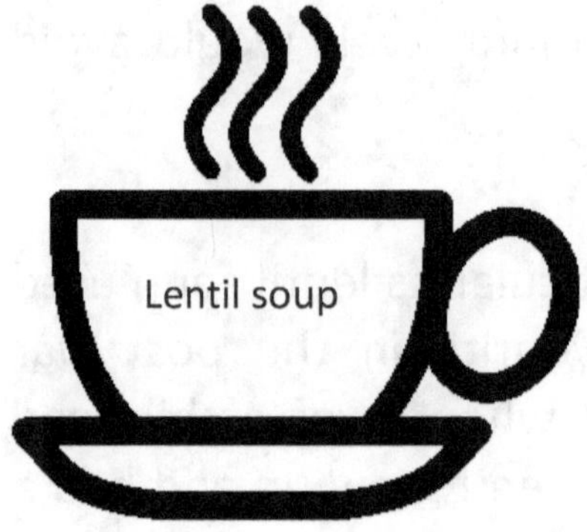

Lentil soup; great sleep inducer, removes anxiety, lessens pain.

I DO NOT recommend taking L-tryptophan in supplement form as there have been some unwanted effects through this route. It is enough to have a diet which adequately addresses any L-tryptophan deficiency.

Nevertheless, for severe chronic pain, it has its uses and is effective although the underlying cause of the pain should be addressed at the same time. High doses of tryptophan can cause constipation so it is effective when diarrhoea is present.

Top dosage is 500mg 3 times a day

Valerian is an herbal product and many insomniacs swear by it. Valerian was a very popular herb in mediaeval times where it was added to soups and stews to flavour them. In truth, valerian smells like stinky socks but its usefulness lies in the mildly sedating properties it has.

Unlike many prescribed medications for insomnia it does not cause brain fog and balance problems.

This is especially good news for the elderly whose balance may not be as good as it used to be.   Further, studies looking at prescribed sleeping pills showed that older people taking a sleeping pill were five times more likely to become confused or forgetful. When we are looking to improve sleep we are also hoping that it will impact positively on overall quality of life, not detract from it.

The recommended dose is 300-600 milligrams daily and this should be continued for a couple of weeks before the effects will be enjoyed. Its use has greater benefit for those with chronic insomnia as opposed to those who are just having a couple of days' difficulty in getting off to sleep.

Natural daylight helps to produce an optimal amount of melatonin. This is because melatonin levels at night are dependent on a complete shutdown of melatonin during the day. The earlier in the day that this occurs the better. Any daylight is better than none but in order to maximise the amount of melatonin production at night, exposure to extremely bright sunlight during the day, is the desirable goal.

We have only to compare the light intensity – which is measured in lux – of that produced in offices (approximately 400 lux) to that of the sun - which is ten times greater during the day - to realise that most of our working life is geared towards producing poor quality sleep.

Most people report that they don't fully wake up in the morning until they have received some 'proper daylight' as opposed to the yellow light emitted by lightest bulbs.

The very elderly housebound, who often complain of poor quality sleep, could very well be victims of the 'yellow light syndrome' since they are hardly ever outside to take advantage of the sun's effects on subsequent melatonin production.

Some groups of people who may suffer from sleep deprivation due to the lack of sunlight are

- the housebound, sick and elderly or even the very young

- office workers

- nurses, teachers, those working underground, shop workers, millworkers, among others

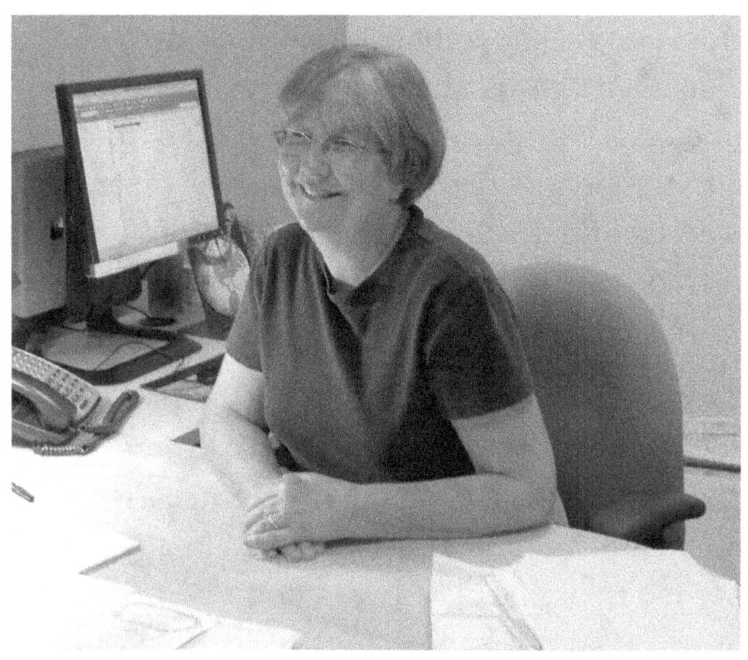

Office workers are not likely to sleep well due to the lack of lux

Don't Take Stimulants before Bedtime (or indeed any nightcap)

It always amazes me that when people say that they cannot sleep - and they run through what they do before bedtime - that they are drinking stimulating nightcaps.

Most people know that caffeine will keep you awake but they probably don't realise how much it can affect an individual's ability to initiate sleep. A cup of coffee, for example, can exert its effects for up to six hours after it has been drunk. In older individual's this could take even longer as our ability to metabolise substances decreases as we age.

However, it is not just the fact that coffee is stimulating that can be the problem; coffee inhibits thiamine and, as we have already learned thiamine is vital for good sleep.

However, coffee is not the only stimulating drink or food. Tea also contains some caffeine but cocoa, often drunk before bedtime, is another beverage which is likely to keep you awake for a number of hours. I have never understood why it is promoted as a bedtime drink. Cocoa, for example, apart from being stimulating is able to destabilise mast cells and release histamine, increasing pain and the risk of heartburn.

Some malted drinks contain high levels of added vitamin B such as pantothenic acid, thiamine, riboflavin, folic acid and niacin. Vitamin B helps release energy but in a controlled gentle way so that the sustained energy released does not cause the blood sugar level drops that so often wake people up.

If a couple of 'healthy' pieces of dark chocolate are eaten at the same time, then it is highly likely that your sleep will be disrupted most of the night. Dark chocolate also contains caffeine but it also contains another sleep preventing chemical called theobromine which is a compound that has caffeine like effects.

Alcohol has been found to interfere with melatonin production. Melatonin is a hormone which helps regulate sleep. While the initial effects of alcohol are to make you feel relaxed and drowsy its later effects are that it will wake you up a lot earlier than you wanted.

 Eating fatty foods late at night has been found to impact on sleep and leads to more fragmented and disrupted sleep as well as contributing to excessive daytime sleepiness.

The impact of fatty foods on preventing good quality sleep was sealed when studies showed that ketogenic diets helped treat patients with narcolepsy – a condition in which the sufferer will fall asleep at any time. That is, ketosis aided wakefulness.

A ketogenic diet is one which is very low in carbohydrates. Normally, glucose is obtained from carbohydrates and provides fuel for muscles and the brain. When the body does not have enough glucose then it burns fat as a fuel in a process called ketosis. It appears that a high fat diet enables a state of wakefulness and, as such, a high fat diet late at night will be disruptive to sleep.

There are many drugs which cause wakefulness and many of these just happen, unfortunately to be medicines which are prescribed to the masses on a regular basis.

As well as caffeine which is found in soft drinks as well as cocoa, tea and coffee. beta blockers such as metoprolol and propranolol and which are prescribed for high blood pressure and heart ailments can also cause insomnia as well as nightmares.

Decongestants such as phenylephrine and pseudoephedrine can make you feel anxious and jittery and disrupt sleep in this way.

Many antidepressants such as Sertraline also impact on the quality of sleep. In fact, the list of drugs which cause sleeplessness is so long that this should be an area of investigation initially when seeking a reason for insomnia.

 The difficulty with many medications, whether over the counter or not, is that while they may treat one condition, it is highly likely that they will cause side effects which will likely need another prescription to deal with them.

The relationship between melatonin and cortisol

Melatonin is, as we have seen, the hormone which regulates the sleep-wake cycle. Cortisol is a steroid hormone that is produced by the adrenal glands. These sit on the top of the kidneys. When cortisol is released into the bloodstream, it can act on many different parts of the body and help it to respond to stress or danger. Cortisol also helps increase the body's metabolism of glucose.

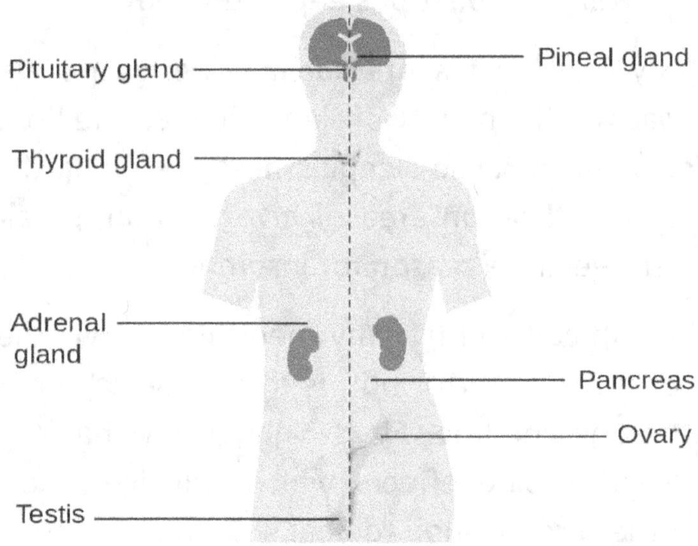

Cortisol is a vital   stress hormone that is designed to aid wakefulness in the morning as well as enable us to cope with danger.

An increase in cortisol also triggers the release of

amino acids from the muscles

 fatty acids into the blood stream as well as

glucose from the liver

 This helps us access an enormous amount of energy should we need it in an emergency.

Modern life does not allow us to burn up this amount of excess energy with intense physical activity. Our lives have become largely sedentary compared to 70 years or so ago

 The elevated levels of hormones continue to impact on the body and stimulate the release of more stress hormones.

When I was teaching and the pupils were coming up to exam time, I used to tell them to run around a lot more than usual just to release all the tension from their bodies.

Many children who find some schoolwork difficult can become agitated and fidgety. They are not being naughty. It is a natural response to the elevated hormones caused by a stressful situation. Punishing a child for this will only worsen the situation.

When people have received worrying news, they can become very agitated and unable to sit still.   This is due to the stress hormones circulating in the body.

Modern day live has been so inculcated into us that it is the norm that we have forgotten that many things which are part and parcel of our lives are stressors. These include

- drinking coffee
- driving
- constant noise
- constant light including the light which surrounds us at night
- too much going on – I find packed supermarkets particularly difficult.

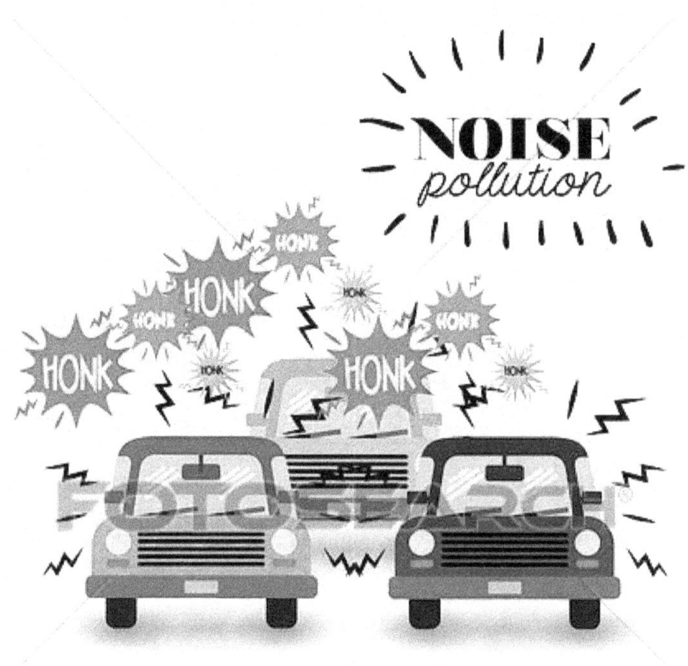

k35093078 www.fotosearch.com

Cortisol has an antagonistic effect on melatonin. As cortisol rises, it correlates with a drop in melatonin and vice versa.

Studies have shown that physical stress decreases pineal melatonin levels at night whereas it increases melatonin production during the day. This is the opposite of what we want.

It is so important to identify the stressors which are impacting on good quality sleep so that adequate amounts of melatonin can be produced.

Nocturia - frequent night time trips to the loo disrupt sleep

This is called nocturia and is a very common cause of sleep loss in older adults especially. Two or more events is associated with daytime tiredness.

Nocturia is often associated with other medical conditions such as a bladder prolapse, disorders of the prostate, heart failure, liver failure, and diabetes, among many others.

Although nocturia always used to be associated with a full bladder, it is also a symptom of sleep apnea. This may seem strange but there are a number of reasons why this might be so. They include:

More difficult to concentrate urine with sleep apnea.

Sleep apnea causes hypoxia. While this is intermittent it still has the potential to cause inflammation due to oxidative stress. Inflammatory episodes can and do cause injury to the endothelium which is associated with vascular permeability and kidney function.

During sleep apnea episodes when the sufferer is holding their breath, then oxygen levels become so low that atrial natriuretic peptide (ANP) will be releases. One of the side effects is that it increases the production of urine.

During the breath holding stage of a sleep apnea episode, the pressure is increased in the abdominal cavity. If you hold your breath this will demonstrate this increased pressure. The increased pressure can make it feel as though you need to urinate.

Nocturia is more common as we age. We produce less of an anti-diuretic hormone which enables us to retain fluid. When this hormone decreases then more urine is produced at night.

Further, the bladder is not able to hold as much as it did when we were younger.

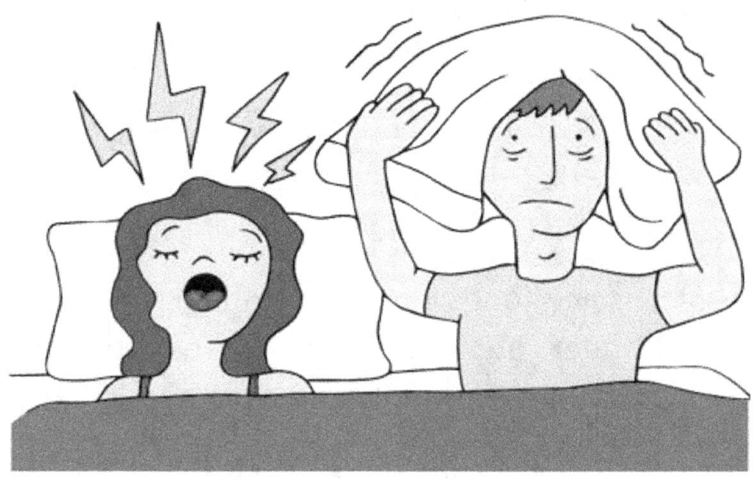

Sleep apnoea can be a risk factor for nocturia not only disturbing your sleep but that of anyone sharing a room with you.:

Potential treatments for nocturia are to limit foods and drink which irritate the bladder or act as diuretics and increase urine output.

Caffeine acts as a diuretic. Alcohol and citrus foods irritate the bladder making it want to empty itself before it is full. These substances are often the culprit in many a frequent night-time trip.

Other bladder irritants are:

- spicy foods
- acidic food like tomatoes
- chocolate
- artificial sweeteners

in fact, spicy foods not only irritate the bowel and bladder but can cause intense burning during bowel movements and an itchy vagina.

Low grade urine infections which haven't been treated promptly can damage the lining of the bladder. This allows irritants in the urine to leak through the coating of the bladder into the interstitium where all the nerves and nerve endings are located.

Once these nerve endings are irritated they initiate a sequence of events which includes the release of substances which act on mast cells which release histamine. It is thought that this causes the bladder to sense frequency and urgency. Repeated insults like the above cause scar tissue to form which is less elastic that it should be thus reducing the capacity of the bladder to hold the amount of urine it was once capable of.

Nevertheless, implementing treatment regimes, which counteract histamine, may be useful for those with nocturia.

These ideally, would be an increase in vitamin C and the inclusion of DAO (olive oil is a good source) and zinc.

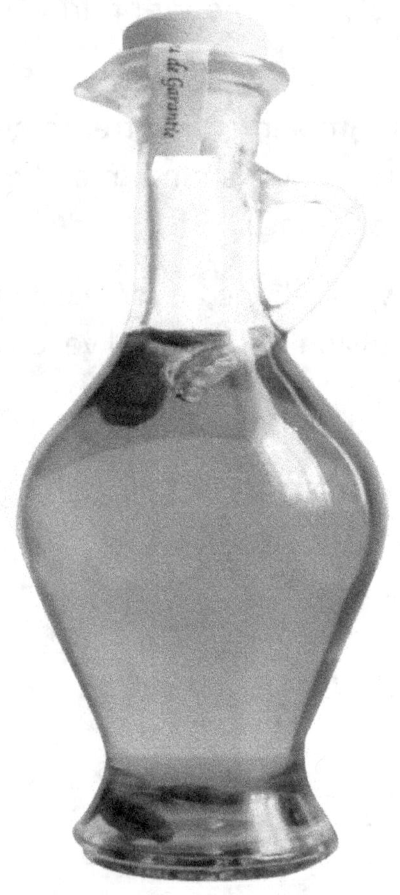

Olive oil enables the increase of diamine oxidase which is a vital enzyme for breaking down histamine.

Excessive heat; mattresses and menopause

We have already learned that the body has to cool a little in order for mechanisms to come into play which enable the initiation of the first stage of sleep.

Mattresses can be the worst culprit for turning what should be a restful night into one of tossing and turning.

The main culprit appears to the mattresses made of memory foam. I understand that they tend to distribute body weight evenly which can relieve joint pain. Indeed, when they were introduced to the market   they were marketed as being suitable for people with hip or shoulder pain.

It also has efficacy for those who are bed bound and at high risk of pressure sores.

However, memory foam retains heat and it is not waterproof.

It gives off a gassy odour

Because it 'gives' when you press on it, then it is difficult to move; turning over can be a problem as the natural spring in a mattress which gives you some leverage isn't there.

While the retention of heat may be useful in winter, it will certainly prevent you from dropping off to sleep in the summer. The extra 'sweat' will remain in the foam and may give off toxic compounds.

It may give rise to allergy symptoms

Memory foam increases the risk of Sudden Infant Death Syndrome.

Even the newer foams such as open cell and gel foams have failed to respond to the need to help the body cool enough for restful sleep.

The fact that moisture can damage the foam by degrading it, is another concern, Humidity and sweat can damage the mattress which is already more expensive than comparable non memory foam mattresses.

If you have ever tried to clean a memory foam mattress – and I have – you will have found it quite a challenge.

In colder weather, the memory foam tends to harden and in warmer weather it tends to become more elastic and less supportive.

Some memory foams have been found to have toxic chemicals such as formaldehyde and benzene in them. These may irritate the airways, skin, eyes and throat.

Clearly, for those with known allergies, this is not a suitable material for a mattress.

Some of the symptoms which may manifest themselves due to the toxicity of the mattresses are:

Headaches

Nausea

Respiratory problems

Brain fog

The risk of Sudden Infant Death Syndrome is entirely due to the fact that carbon dioxide gets trapped in the foam

Research has also shown that when lungs are irritated by toxic substances then it can reduce the airflow by approximately 20%

Clearly, there are many reasons why a memory foam mattress and pillows may not be the best way forward if you want to be assured of a good night's sleep.

The menopause is a rite of passage which tends to disrupt many women's sleep due to the dreaded hot flashes.

Hot flashes occur when there is decrease in the hormone oestrogen. When oestrogen levels drop then other hormones, which impact on the hypothalamus are released causing the body's temperature to fluctuate.

Although this appears to be a fairly innocuous process, it does cause a great deal of misery for women when it disrupts their sleep patterns many times a night.

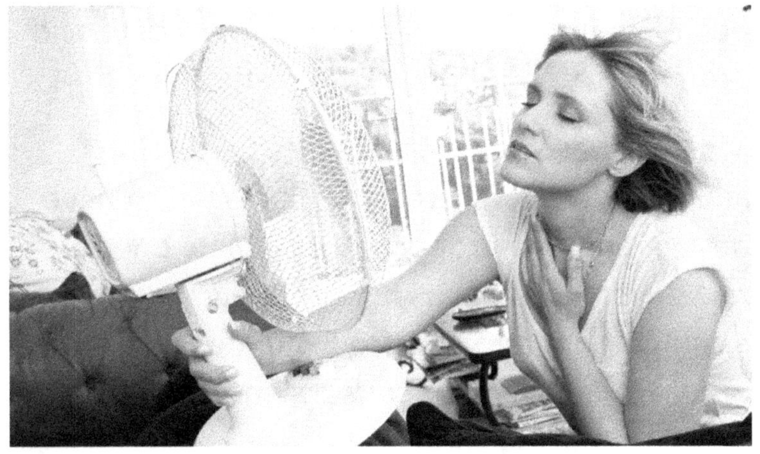

Menopausal hot flushes are disruptive during the day and during attempts to sleep

The time period for hot flashes and night sweats to occur tends to be approximately four years although some people experience them for decades and others only suffer intermittently or tend to get 'overheated' more than others.

Many menopausal women start sleeping with the windows open for the first time in their lives.

Hormone replacement therapy is effective but not all women want to go down that route and prefer to try something more natural.

Most of these natural remedies tend to be along the lives of increasing plants which have oestrogenic like properties. The main ones are red clover; soya beans are probably the most popular food item to introduce into the diet in order to reduce menopausal symptoms.

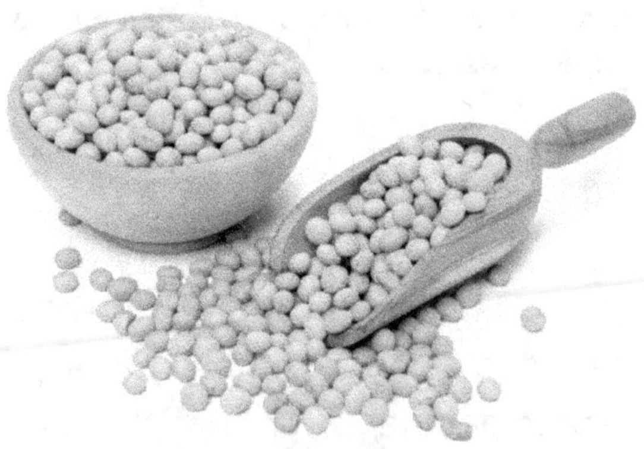

Soya beans have oestrogen like qualities

Vitamin C – which is hardly ever mentioned as being able to alleviate hot flashes – is able to help with hormone balance.

Vitamin C is linked to higher progesterone levels and lower follicle stimulating hormone levels. These are associated with a good balance of hormones.

Many women will testify that during periods of stress that hot flashes become worse. Vitamin C is vital in the proper functioning of the adrenal glands. Pantothenic acid – vitamin B5- is also useful in this respect.

The amino acid, glycine also affects oestrogen and helps to build bone when the menopause is a time when bone tends to become less dense.

Glycine also helps to reduce adipogenesis, the synthesis of fat which will also help to reduce body temperature.

Further, dose dependent decreases in body temperature occur with glycine. What a marvellous amino acid; the smallest, yes, but it packs a powerful punch.

Supplement wise no more than 3g should be taken daily but dietary glycine increase is probably the best way forward to begin with.

As we have already seen, glycine is found in bone broth and gelatinous type foods like:

Jelly

Wine gums (made with gelatine)

Slow cooked meats like brisket

All meats

Fish

Hard cheeses

Seeds

Beas

Cabbage

Mushrooms

The cooling effect that glycine produce is down to increases in blood flow to the skin

In an article entitled

Severity of hot flushes is inversely associated with dietary intake of vitamin B6 and oily fish

Investigations into the associations between vasomotor symptoms and nutrients were undertaken.

262 women from ages of 40-65 years participated and considered in the light of the Menopausal Health-Related Quality of life Questionnaire. In addition, a self-administered Diet History Questionnaire aided the researchers to find potential associations.

43 nutrients were included; adjustments were made for factors such as body mass index.

The conclusion drawn was that there was a significant inverse relationship   between menopausal symptoms and oily fish and vitamin B6.

It appears that omega-3 fatty acids in conjunction with moderate exercise is associated with higher levels of oestrogen

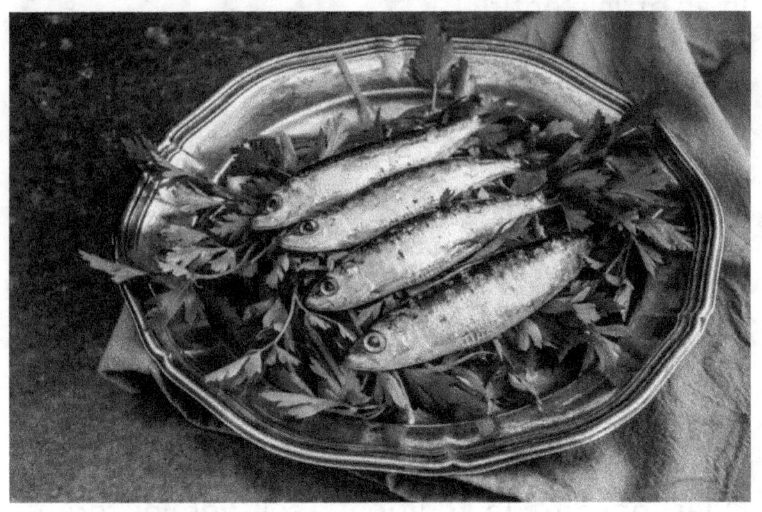

Sardines are full of omega 3 fatty acids

Finally, we should not forget boron, a mineral which is only found in plant based foods but is required to   help the absorption of both testosterone and oestrogen.

There is a wealth of research of the benefits of boron for menopausal women but very little, if any reaches the patient from the doctor's surgery.

Boron, as well as helping to increase oestrogen levels is a powerful anti-inflammatory to the extent that it reduces pain better than most over the counter and prescription medications prescribed for inflammation; this without damaging the stomach lining either.

Good sources of boron include:

Raisins

Prunes

Apples

Pears

Grapes

Peaches

Spinach

kale

legumes

nuts

    whole grains
potatoes,
cider
beer

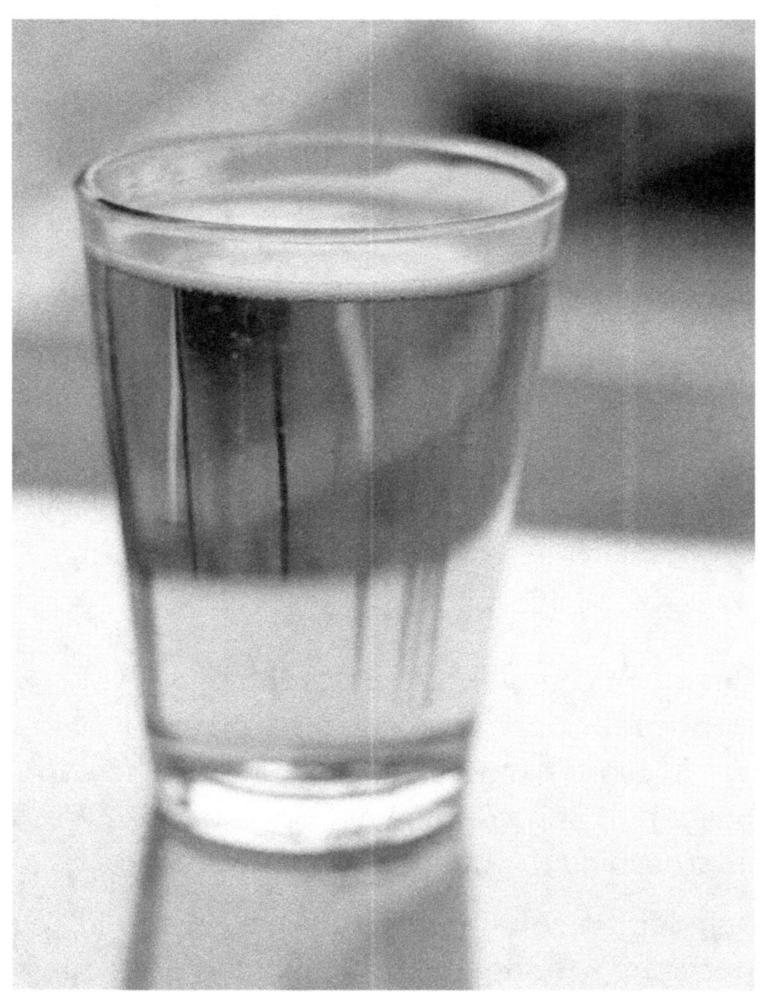

Beer is a good source of boron.

The amount of boron in plants can vary depending on the type of plant and the amount of boron in the soil. The average person's diet contains 1.5–3 milligrams of boron per day.

Boron is a trace mineral that may help with bone health. While it's generally safe for most people, large amounts can be harmful. You should consult your doctor before taking supplements.

Vitamin B complex also helps the body synthesise oestrogen and also enables it to use it, too. I cannot repeat oft enough how the B vitamins appear to be deficient in those approaching the menopause and beyond.

 In addition, Vitamin D acts as a secosteroid - a hormone - in the body and, like the B vitamins helps in the synthesis of oestrogen production.

A high proportion of the population is deficient in many nutrients anyway so it is no surprise that as the ability to absorb nutrients lessens that   distressing symptoms will manifest themselves but the good news is that they can be reduced to manageable levels or eliminated altogether.

FINAL THOUGHTS

When we look at many of the potential causes of poor sleep we find that many are related to our way of life – the blue light radiating from screens, the constant light from streetlights, noise pollution and our diets.

Unfortunately, light and noise have become such a major part of our lives that we do not realise the impact they are having on our quality of sleep.

We do not associate working in an office with a lack of production of melatonin at night due to unsatisfactory light levels.

Snatching a rushed coffee has become part and parcel of our life. If we could see the impact that excess levels of cortisol have on our bodies and minds then we might just do something about it but that association rarely, if ever, is made.

As a helpful exercise it might be useful to jot down the stressors which are affecting the quality of sleep as you go through the book whether it is that last glass of wine before you go to bed to help relax you or the street light which allows a chink of light into your bedroom or, indeed, many of the others mentioned in this book. You might be surprised at how many that there are.

Of course, they all need to be eliminated. It is no use saying 'Well, I've always drunk three cups of coffee a day and it never did me any harm.' Coffee apart from containing caffeine also inhibits vitamin B1, a vitamin which is vital for prolonged and refreshing sleep.

For those who are younger, that is as it may be but as you get older the impact of those stressors exerts a far greater effect than it is likely to have done when you were younger so it is worth eliminating them all and then introducing known potential stressors to see which ones aren't causing the problem. Each individual is unique and furthermore, requirements change over time.

However, sleep quality is also impacted by diet and even by choice of mattress. We haven't even touched on other stresses such as those found in relationship problems. While it might be our right to a good night's sleep,

 good sleep hygiene must be worked at and adhered to. It is no good thinking that one late night coffee while working at the screen won't harm, it will, just as a poor diet will.

The body runs on good nutrition, exercise and rest.

There is no other formula.

Thank you for purchasing this book. Every time a book is purchased, a donation is made to one of the charities I am currently supporting. These can be found on my author's website. See below.

Other Health Related Books by the Author

- **The Reluctant Bowel**
- **A Weighty Issue**
- **Sleep, Perchance to Dream**
- **The Journey: EDS and chronic pain**
- **The MND diet: using nutrition to slow down the progress of neurodegeneration**
- **A Necessary Sorrow**
- **Taking another Road: Pain: its causes and what can be done about it**
- **The incontinence Diet**
- **Allergies and Intolerances**
- **The Parkinson's Disease diet**
- **And many more**

These can be found here on the author's page

https://www.amazon.co.uk/-/e/B07BPQZ5CD

You may also be interested in the semi-autobiographical trilogy of the authors life found in these three books

- The Prejudged
- Where the Blackbird Never Sings
- A Summer's Symphony

And the author's children's books

- Fanny and Victorian Jack
- Fanny and the Gamekeeper's Cottage